THE MENOPAUSE MONOLOGUES

Real experiences by real women

(and a few men!)

Compiled by Harriet Powell

Cover and illustrations by M.R. Goodwin

All contributors' names have been changed unless otherwise requested.

First Printing 2019

The Little Taboo Press

ISBN 978-1-9161391-0-7

Introduction

This time last year I was driving to work and listening to the radio when *Woman's Hour* came on. It was Menopause Week, and Radio 4 had teamed up with Radio Sheffield to cover as many aspects of the menopause as they could over five days. Today the general public was to take to the air.

Woman after woman phoned into the programme, and in the end I had to pull over so I could listen properly. I was, to say the least, shocked. Was the menopause really still such a taboo subject? Were people not able to talk freely about it at work, with their partners and children, with their friends?

The germ of an idea took root in my head, and that evening I began to email friends – and friends of friends – to see if they would consider sending me their 'stories': their own personal experiences of the menopause. I even asked a few men for their takes.

This is the result. I haven't done much editing: I think the no holds barred approach is the best. I hope you'll find it as moving, informative and entertaining as I do. My greatest wish is that it helps to get us all talking about something which half the population will go through (and many of the other half will experience second-hand).

Happy reading!

The Women

Amber's story

I'm taking it personally. I have no choice: my menopause is like no one else's. Even though it is universal to women, no two experiences can be the same. Oh, how hearteningly unique my menopause is to me.

I'm a late bloomer in every way: with my sexuality (not until my twenties); with marriage (mid-thirties); with falling in love good and proper (mid-forties). Also by my forties I felt I finally had a certain dancing relationship with my career, a reasonable sense of self and a handle on my health and fitness. And then, just before the bell-toll of my 50th birthday, there came the sudden end to a loving relationship. It seemed to precipitate me into a mysterious chain of poor health. It was grief, but it was also the menopause arriving. Migraines hit, my digestion could be toppled over one bread roll, my immunity seemed to labour under a system that was more stressed than I had stress with which to justify it. Oh, and hot flushes. My broiled face and that sudden 'glow' that advertised to the world that, yup, over the hill was where I was rolling.

What a journey is womanhood. We have grappled with periods and, for some, pregnancy, childbirth and breast-feeding. Our bodies have belonged to rhythms and cycles beyond our control. We have been subjected to incredible physical and emotional change. Now, as older women, we have arrived at a time of life that we might dare call Ours. But that ole gangster Menopause is waiting for us. And even though the big M is universal and half the population is going to go through it in some form or other, we so often seem to keep it to ourselves. It's our shameful secret. We are no longer viable as child-bearers, we can no longer hope to own a youthful air. We have no choice but to say it's over rover: no one can pretend I'm fecund anymore.

Then there's the thrashing around in bed at night, seeking that sweet position that might just be comfortable. I mean, what kind of revenge is that?

I know that my own hormonal experience is quite mild compared to some. My least favourite symptom has been the flushes, which also brought an intense pressure in the head and a pounding heart. They were striking maybe four times an hour. After trying a plethora of different herbal and vitamin tablets, I eventually discovered a herbal combination that helped. But then there is the other troubling health surprise: the strain on my liver and digestion. I don't know for sure what's causing it, and unless I pay to have a diagnosis, I suppose it will remain a mystery.

However, I'm happy to report that I did have a period (excuse the pun) of 'remission' from my menopausal symptoms and was truly grateful for the time off. And when they started again, they were easier to handle.

I hear it can be ten years before it's all properly over. Don't they give you that for murder? Who knows when it's finished, so maybe we should all open up about it in the meantime and raise a glass (of herbal tea) to the Mystery of Menopause.

Mo's story

One of the strangest things to have struck me about this menopause malarkey is how disproportionately weepy I become when I listen to, or read about, other people talking about it! Basically, I become emotional and upset about just how very emotional and upsetting it can all be.

I mention this because I am currently listening to Radio 4's *Woman's Hour,* during which the menopause is being discussed (it is Menopause Week – hurrah!) and, of course, I am crying. Why? I can't really tell you, and that's the problem. My emotions are unreliable, and I'm not entirely sure whether I'm going to be in a screaming fury, weeping morosely, or a sunny delight from one minute to the next. And this is all, apparently, because I am perimenopausal.

For me it started fairly early, at the age of 39. Not long before my 40th birthday, I started experiencing hot flushes. It took a while to suss out that these might be linked to the menopause: after all, I was still in my thirties and had only recently suffered a miscarriage. I assumed that, since I had managed to become pregnant (for once without any extra fertility intervention) only a couple of months earlier, my ovaries and hormones, though unreliable, were still functioning.

It turns out that they were, but very sporadically.

It also explained why it had been so hard for me to become pregnant over the previous years – because apparently this perimenopausal phase can start gradually, and far earlier than we might all assume.

I realise now that in my thirties I had been drifting towards perimenopause with my exceedingly irregular periods, and by the age of 39, I was wafting in and out of it every few months; for three months I might experience the frequent hideousness of hot flushes and then suddenly they'd be gone. Then a few months later they'd be back with a vengeance.

I could think of only one explanation for these hot flushes, so I went to the doctor to ask whether he thought I might be starting the menopause. He thought it unlikely as I was relatively young, but the blood tests came back pretty conclusive: it seemed that I had indeed arrived at that unwelcome milestone.

This was not good news. I had wanted at least a second child – my first (and only) having been born a year and a half earlier through IVF – but now this looked increasingly unlikely. This was a massive blow and an emotional crash all of its own, but the menopause itself brought other horrors. I felt old. Didn't the menopause make me middle-aged or past-it? And the hot flushes were horrendous – the sudden need to throw myself into a fridge as that red-hot sensation crept over my whole body became a far too regular part of daily life, to the extent that I felt I had to explain myself whenever my face was suffused with an attractive shade of tomato. And let's face it, most people don't really want to be drawn into a conversation about hot flushes. At night they were almost unbearable: hours were spent alternately throwing off all the covers and then grabbing them back again when the sweat dried, leaving me shivering between each unpleasant, fiery bout.

Because of the night sweats, I was also, of course, tired. But I didn't really realise it. So I was ratty. A lot of the time. I guess I should have been used to being emotionally unpredictable by this stage. During the preceding five years I had been riding the Hormone Rollercoaster: misery at not becoming pregnant; hormonal mood swings on various, unpleasant fertility drugs; a miscarriage; the highs and lows of IVF; pregnancy itself; post-natal depression; another miscarriage. And now the menopause. And of course, it could also be hard to elicit sympathy from those closest to me when I spent so much of the time being irritable, cross or down.

And that's the awful thing. I couldn't remember whether I had always been like this or whether it was the result of hormonal imbalance. At times I felt like I had become somebody I didn't recognise. I still do a lot of the time, because I'm not through this yet.

I resisted HRT for a couple of years – I'm not really sure why – but when the GP appealed to my vanity by explaining that feeding fake versions of oestrogen and progesterone back into my body would help stave off those additional symptoms brought on by menopause such as dry, crepe-like skin, brittle hair and nails, I decided to go for it. After all, I was still only 42.

It was recommended that I didn't take pills because I'd suffered migraines in the past, meaning that the risk of blood clots and stroke would have been slightly increased. I was therefore prescribed patches, which apparently carry less risk.

Patches. Another nightmare. I have this weird foible which means I can't stand things stuck to my skin – the Rizla game is torture for me and I can't even bear to have a phone number written on my hand – so this was going to be tough: a large sticky square constantly stuck to my inner thigh or butt cheek. I also realised that when it came to summer and swimming costumes I would have to be very careful about positioning: patches aren't the most glamorous of accessories and certainly not something I fancied showing off. But needs must, so I forced myself to wear them, and gradually they became routine. And hallelujah, the flushes disappeared! And with them, the night sweats. If nothing else, this was excellent news. The mere absence of these was a thrill for a while and I thanked heaven for HRT.

I had also been holding out for a mood (or preferably whole personality) transplant as another happy side effect but I can't really say whether my general demeanour improved whilst on these patches. It may have done slightly.

The downside of the patches was that they effectively put me back into a regular menstrual cycle, so while the only upside of the perimenopause had been that periods only arrived once or twice a year, now I was back to having them every month. And that meant I didn't really know what was going on with my body naturally. If I stayed on HRT, how on earth would I know when I had finally gone through the menopause, given that this is defined as when you have gone a whole year without a period?

Well, apparently you have to guess! And then try a different type of HRT in the hope this will suit your body, even though you don't know what it would actually be doing if left to its own devices. So, after two years, the doctor called me in to do an assessment of my HRT needs and suggested that I move onto a different variety. The idea was that whereas before, the HRT had given me oestrogen through the whole month and then progesterone towards the end of it (ie to bring on a period and mimic a menstrual cycle), this new prescription would drip-feed me both hormones (substitutes) in lesser quantities but throughout the entire month. I shouldn't have any bleeds either.

Sounded good. Wasn't.

Before, I had had healthy bouts of grumpiness – effectively what felt like your average PMT at the end of every month, but now I was a she-devil *all the time.* It was horrendous. I shouted a lot, sobbed a lot, and sometimes felt like screaming. I probably would have if I'd lived on top of a hill miles from anywhere, rather than in a terraced town house on the other side of the wall from a charming, genteel and self-contained widow.

It didn't take long to work out that this whole new level of hormonal horribilis had coincided with the new HRT patches I was on. So back to the doctor I went.

This time I was presented with a truck-load of boring and unappealing options: go back to the previous HRT and remain totally oblivious to the natural rhythms of my unpredictable body; try a different one; stay on this one for longer.

I decided at this point to give up on all HRT, even at the risk of drier, older skin and more brittle, stringier hair. Vanity be damned. I wanted to know what was going on and hoped that in a year I might be through it, and so I went cold turkey.

It was a good decision – but I'm not through it yet. After six months, I had a period out-of-the-blue, which was rather frustrating. So I guess my body hasn't totally given up on all of its oestrogen yet. The flushes came back too. As soon as the first one crept over me, I felt marginally depressed – and far more so after numerous sleepless nights.

I experimented with a few natural supplements, including a cream containing bio-identical hormones. Weirdly, it seemed to work on the flushes, even though there's no real evidence for its efficacy – but it gave me a monthly bleed and I couldn't be bothered to keep ordering it online in time.

I also tried black cohosh and St John's Wort but started to suffer headaches. I wasn't sure which of these was the culprit but didn't fancy going through another week or two of pain just to figure it out. They didn't do anything particularly useful anyway.

What I really want now is to find someone who can tailor some bio-identical hormones to me. My GP knew nothing about this, but I have spoken to one or two people who do. No one yet has been able to take the necessary blood samples and prescribe accordingly. But I think this is the way forward.

I have been in a no-flush zone for the past three months, which probably explains why the bleed happened. But even as I type, a warmish flush has just stolen over me, so perhaps I am about to re-enter the world of the hot. Who knows? Unpredictable, this menopause.

I'm 46 now and getting a bit bored with it all. What I do know is that I want to get past it. I'm through with worrying about feeling old, but I'm very aware that I need to be more vigilant in the measures I take to feel – and look – my best. Yes, vanity again. It really sucks that the menopause brings physical symptoms of ageing, especially if you are someone who got there early.

There are other aspects which I find challenging and troubling, such as the fact that during the menopause women feel hungrier, but their bodies are less able to metabolise food as quickly as they once did, so even to maintain their weight, they should eat less. Which is hard when their bodies are telling them they want more. Clearly, I need to exercise greater self-control, but there are some days when only chocolate will take away these blues…

I'm told there are some who come out the other side of the menopause superwomen. They get through this bit and then suddenly: athletes, achievers, beauties, brainboxes all. Please let that be me. It would make such a nice change from the muddle-headed, crotchety, sometimes-nice-but-sometimes-not, sweaty, slightly lardy woman I feel I've been for too long. So, bring on the good stuff, Mother Nature: I'm ready to move on.

Rosa's story

I suspect that my experience is exceptional, but – hand-on-heart – I really do have to say: "Menopause? What menopause?" A little early maybe (late forties?), as I was an ovary down following what a quick search tells me was an 'oophorectomy' (fabulous word) several years before, but I found myself postmenopausal without really having taken on board that anything had happened.

The only clue was that I no longer had to deal with the nuisance and pain of periods. In fact it wasn't until I was asked at my triennial smear test, "When was your last period?" that I realised I hadn't had one for at least eighteen months.

It wasn't that I'd had a particularly easy time over the previous twenty-five years either: it was double-strength ibuprofen and super-plus everything all the way. I guess I was just fortunate in my genes. My mother always said she never noticed anything either, although my older sisters have a different tale to tell.

So what more can I say but…lucky, lucky me!

Lara's story

The problem with being menopausal – or at least perimenopausal – is that the symptoms seem to change all the time. The physical ones are easy to identify, but the emotional ones are much harder.

The clearest physical sign for me was the increasingly irregular nature of my periods, from about the age of 45. After having my children, I settled into a reasonably regular cycle, but now I go long stretches between bleeds. At first this was a cue for panic: was another baby about to make an appearance? When I do have a period, it either goes on for ages in a half-hearted sort of way or it is short-lived but dramatic. On one memorable occasion I was delivering a class to a group of Year 10 boys – dressed, of course, in a new pair of pale blue jeans – when all hell broke loose: not an experience I ever wish to repeat.

About a year ago I had five solid months of night sweats. Although they interrupted my sleep, they were manageable once I'd removed the duvet, but I can't say I'm looking forward to their inevitable return. I also suffer from very tender breasts, so tender it often hurts just to take off my bra. When my periods were regular, my breasts were often sore before a bleed, so maybe I'm prone to it.

I wage a constant battle with my figure. I've always been quite slim, and in the past, my weight was easy to maintain. Now it's down to sheer willpower, together with regular swimming and walking. I could very easily balloon. I no longer have any tolerance for alcohol. Also, for about the last three years I have woken up feeling stiff and achy. Sometimes very stiff and achy. The feeling eases once I've got moving. Oh, and the back of my neck is permanently itchy. Figure that one out.

I've noticed a definite change in my libido over the past couple of years. Sex still happens quite a lot, and once initiated I always enjoy it, but I've lost my drive to dive between the sheets at every opportunity. I think it's important to make time for it and just accept it won't be as spontaneous as before. At least I'm not yet suffering from vaginal dryness, but if it *does* strike, a friend of mine has pointed me in the direction of a good lubricant.

People joke about perimenopausal brain fog. Well, in my experience it's no laughing matter. It's one thing to forget what you came upstairs for, but quite another then to go back downstairs, remember what it was, trek back upstairs and forget *again*. In a similar vein, I forget people's names and frequently forget where I have parked the car. I once stood at the sink washing up a casserole dish, completely unable to dredge from my mind the word 'casserole'. It is hugely scary. If you suffer from perimenopausal brain fog and crave to know you're normal, I urge you to read *How Hard Can It Be?* by Allison Pearson. Let's just say I could seriously do with a Roy in my life.

I've always been anxious and irritable (or worse) before a period: classic PMT, I suppose. But I think it's important to think carefully before putting any increased irritability at this stage of life simply down to being perimenopausal. I had a great chat with one of my GPs about this recently: all mine are truly worth their weight in gold. So many things are changing for me right now: two of my children are university age and leaving home, and the other two are just coming into their teenage years. They all still need me, but not in such a physical and time-consuming way as they did when they were younger, and I can definitely sense new opportunities and excitement – both in my work life and more generally – around the corner. Time for myself again. And the more I taste this newfound freedom, the more I want of it. When I don't get enough, I get irritable, and because my periods are all over the place, it's impossible to know whether it's hormones that are to blame, or my changing circumstances. It's probably a combination of both.

As things stand, I plan to get through the menopause without medication. I've never been good with drugs of any kind: ibuprofen upsets my stomach, antihistamines send me straight to sleep and contraceptive pills mess with my mood and make me feel sick. I'm a strictly three-paracetamols-a-year kind of girl. Having said that, if my symptoms get worse, my mind isn't entirely shut to possibilities. I'd just rather work with nature if I can.

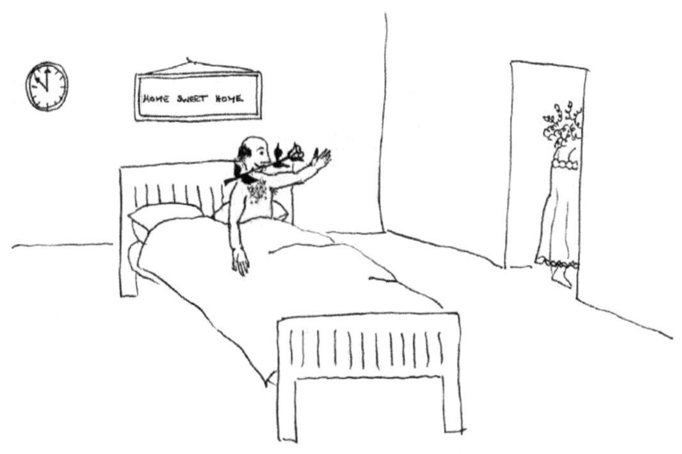

Millie's story

For the first forty years of my life I was too cold. As a small child I'd shiver on the beach, wrapped in a towel while everyone else enjoyed the sun. I'd wear gloves indoors and boil myself in hot baths to try and maintain some kind of normal body temperature. My mum bought me a sort of sleeping-bag I could wear while I was doing my homework. I was part-girl, part-lizard: I needed external forces to warm me up.

When I moved in with my husband (to a caravan with a hole in the roof and a hole in the floor), I made two stipulations: that he complain neither about the phone bill nor the heating. I spent most evenings chatting to pals while huddled in front of a gas fire wearing my coat. I wore even more clothes to bed, and always a woolly hat. It was so cold the loo water would freeze solid: even a hot wee couldn't always break through the thick ice. Romantic, eh?

Then something happened.

For about the last ten years, I've been too hot and getting progressively hotter – especially in bed. (I'm talking temperature here: I wouldn't *dream* of commenting on any other kind of hotness, though I will say that confidence comes with age.) So I now sleep naked under a four-tog duvet with the window open, even in the depths of winter. My confused other-half is the one in pyjamas with his socks on. I changed my mattress because I was convinced it was making me hot. Several hundred pounds later and I'm still poking my legs out of the covers, desperately seeking a cold patch and facing the reality that the adjusted thermostat is actually inside me. Being a woman of a certain age, that raises the inevitable question: is it the menopause?

I have no idea, and that's because of a magic plastic anchor nestled in my womb: the Mirena coil – or the Miracoil, as I like to call it. It's a fabulous thing, and it means that I only have to think about contraception once every five years. It also means I haven't had a period for fifteen years, which makes it rather tricky to tell if they've become irregular.

Let me be clear. I'm not that bothered. And that's because of something that happened nearly two decades ago.

Husband and I had settled into life on a new farm. We'd sold our house to buy a bit of land and were living in a caravan (again). We were happy, our daughter had settled easily into her new school, we were doing what we wanted, for ourselves. Husband never once complained about the heating or the phone bill and all was well. Then I started to feel nauseous. My breasts were sore, my belly swollen. I had all the signs of pregnancy and I panicked.

It wasn't that I didn't want another child. I didn't want another *labour.* Having my daughter had shredded my insides and afterwards I had required extensive repair surgery, front and back, to put my innards back where they should be. Another birth would likely lead to devastating injuries and it terrified me. Just in case, I did a pregnancy test, even though I was on the pill and diligent about taking it. I was showing signs of serious hormonal activity and what else could it be?

The test was negative.

I went to my doctor. She did a pregnancy test too, just in case. It was also negative. So what was my crazy body doing? The doctor thought I might be having an early menopause. She asked me to come back in for hormone tests the next time I had a period. I found myself stricken with an incomprehensible grief. I might have decided I was never giving birth again, but faced with the reality of never having another child – of having the choice taken away from me – it was devastating.

The wait for my next period to arrive, so I could have the hormone tests that would confirm the end of my fertility, was miserable. Nothing happened. No period arrived. But my belly continued to swell. I did one more pregnancy test, *just in case.* A pale blue line appeared. I wasn't having an early menopause. I was having a baby. The relief, the joy, was overwhelming. I was scared as well but I also knew I wanted the baby like nothing I'd ever wanted before.

I won't give you the full birth story but suffice to say, my body was still rubbish at pushing big baby heads out of a tiny hole. This time though, I was better informed and instead of spending twenty-six hours ripping myself to shreds, my son was born by C-section. The radio was on, they unzipped me and handed me my boy. Within moments, he was having his first feed. I wouldn't change a thing about his arrival, but I was advised it probably wasn't wise to have another baby, given how rubbish I was at birthing them. That's how the Miracoil took residence, and bloody marvellous it's been too.

Roll on nearly twenty years…was that coil masking the menopause? Or was my super-heated body caused by something else? With no periods, how was I supposed to work it out? I asked Dr Internet. Did I have any of the symptoms?

Hot flushes: I'm just hot all the time, but maybe there are other reasons for that. I do a lot more sport than I did in my thirties, partly because I finally gave in to a competitive streak that I'd denied for most of my adult life, and partly to offset the weight that had crept on after I'd had my children. I also went on a low carb diet and shed two and a half stone. Was that it? Does improving your muscle to fat ratio make you hotter? According to my research, it doesn't.

Difficulty sleeping: Well, yes, obviously. I'm too flipping hot to sleep. I lie awake writing chapters in my head so I'm not wasting the time as the clock nudges 3am. But then I've never been a good sleeper. When I was young it was down to horror stories: I was pretty much permanently too terrified to close my eyes. Then I had my daughter, now a wonderful young woman, but as far as I know, someone who has *never* slept through the night. Listening out for crying/walking/sleepless children became a default night time status I've never recovered from.

Loss of libido: Possibly. I still look at my other half and want to tear his clothes off pretty much most of the time, but in recent years, that urge has subsided a bit. I still, you know, *would* but… I'm also happy to curl up with a glass of wine and a good book. The edge has been taken off my need and that is kind of fine. More convenient in a way because honestly, I think I wore my husband out. So is that a symptom or am I just more knackered because I'm older and insanely busy?

Headaches: Nope, thank goodness.

Joint pain: I'm 50 and trying to qualify to fence for my country: obviously I have joint pain.

Wee infections: Got those all the time when I was younger, much improved now.

Vaginal dryness: ALRIGHT. You've got me. This is a thing. And it's horrible, but solvable. There are lubricants out there, not just for this but that are designed to increase your sexual pleasure – and lo! They actually work. I'd never have discovered that secret if I hadn't gone out looking.

Out of seven usual symptoms, I've got one definite, two maybes and four thank-god-nots. So I still don't know if I'm going through the menopause. It is kind of like being thirteen when everyone else has got their period and you are still waiting, because honestly, I'm happy to join this new generational sisterhood. It means I've made it this far. I'm still alive, and it feels pretty fantastic. Plus there are compensations: the lubricants are really fun and I'm saving so much money on the heating.

Sandy's story

I started the menopause when I was 52. I noticed my periods became irregular, with longer and longer gaps between each one. They also became lighter. I was about 54 when they stopped altogether. At the same time, I began to get night sweats and hot flushes. The night sweats would occur in bouts, two or three times a week, with gaps of several weeks in-between. I would wake up in the middle of the night drenched in sweat and have to change my nightie. Everything had to be 100% cotton. I couldn't bear anything man-made, like polyester. On some occasions the sheets would be soaked too. Over a period of about three or four years, this gradually decreased.

Hot flushes were awful, especially when they occurred in public. From an early age I tended to blush very easily and because I am fair-skinned, hot flushes made me look like a lobster. I would usually have a warning of feeling a bit uncomfortable, and then the heat and redness would start across my upper chest and spread gradually up my neck and into my face and scalp. This was accompanied by feeling hot, prickly and sweaty and I often had beads of sweat on my upper lip. This would last only a few minutes, but often felt much longer.

I was lucky enough to work in a hospital with two lovely nurses who were a similar age to me, and we suffered together. In fact, we had a code! If you felt a hot flush coming on during a busy outpatient clinic, you would murmur, "I have to see Dr Broadbent," and then you could disappear to the loo for five minutes until it subsided. One of the good things about working in the eye department was that a lot of the examinations took place in a dark or semi-dark room, with bright lights shining in the patients' eyes, so if a hot flush started you could just spend an extra minute or so on the slit lamp until the tell-tale signs eased. (Dr Broadbent was very useful throughout my medical career: he was always a great excuse when I had morning sickness and had to retch down the loo for a while.)

I found hot flushes were generally worse after alcohol and spicy food. They gradually petered out, but I still get the occasional one (maybe two per year) aged 74!

Sasha's story

My ears are on fire!

That's not something you expect to find yourself thinking at the ripe old age of forty-nine-and-three-quarters. I'd heard about hot flushes, but so far mine appear to have confined themselves to the two organs on either side of my head. Weird! The fire is accompanied by a fetching shade of somewhere between puce and scarlet. And since I keep my hair very short (yes, it's starting to thin – if I were to try and grow it, I would definitely be sporting the wispy, frizzy look), I now find myself resembling something rather like a garden gnome.

As of yet, I'm not deep in the throes of The Change. 'Time-of-the-month' is still very much a feature of my life, but no longer a regular one. It's now more a case of 'Time-of-whenever-the-heck-it-feels-like-it'. So, almost as though I had reverted to teenagehood, these days I'm forced to carry around the necessary gear All The Time, on the offchance. And not only is it a case of *whenever*, it's also *whatever* – anything from a trickle to a flood, and lasting from twenty-four hours to five days. Oh, and I'm starting to get the odd zit too: terrific.

I have definitely detected signs of 'mid-life crisis', with all the usual clichés (What have I done with my life?... Help, I have less time left on this earth than I've already spent on it!... Lord, please don't let me turn into my aged parents… Lord, please don't let me die from the same hideous ailments as my aged parents… And the latest item on my bucket list (no longer simply a 'to do' list) is…), but at least I'm aware that I'm doing it and that it's mainly down to hormones.

There are upsides to all of this. Firstly, I have decided that the best way of dealing with the menopause is to try and get reasonably fit. Rather than heading for the gym, I have taken up early-morning swimming, and boy do I feel better for it! I can't quite shift the middle-aged spread which is settling around my midriff, but the rest of me is now reasonably taut. And I feel sure that keeping it that way will have a positive, mitigating effect on whatever physical horrors Mother Nature decides to hurl at me next.

The other positive thing (please, oh please, let it last!) is really significant to my health and well-being. I have had some form of migraine all my adult life. It is most definitely hormone-related, and it has morphed over the years from the usual, classic, appalling headache accompanied by intolerance of any form of light or sound, to the aura which renders one temporarily sight-impaired and is followed by a general feeling of fatigue, right through to three-day bouts of dizziness and vomiting – all the symptoms of a nasty virus, minus the raging temperature – culminating in several days of feeling like one is swimming through treacle. But now I only get an aura about once a week, accompanied by an overwhelming desire to eat something carb-laden at the earliest opportunity, and then a general feeling of tiredness for a few hours or so. That is a huge improvement on the three-day horrors which have stalked me for the past few years. If this is the shape of things to come…well, I can live with it.

Elizabeth's story

I think the menopause is something women should look forward to, albeit with some apprehension. It was a subject my mother never mentioned, but then neither did she explain periods.

I was relieved to experience a rapid and early menopause. My cycle, unless medically organised, spanned twenty-one days, and at around the age of 42 my periods started to peter out. I suppose I might have had to put up with a few hot flushes, but that was it.

Many of my friends, and also my elder daughter, have since told me how extraordinarily lucky I was: by 43 or 44 it was all over.

It can be as painless as that, and if it's not, a sympathetic doctor can provide some hope. Don't suffer in silence.

Imogen's story

I have been on my menopausal journey since I was 48, and am now 60. Fingers crossed I'm nearly done...

There have, in fact, been many happy and exciting times during my menopause, and I'd like to give a passing wave to the great surge of energy, intellectual awakening and personal awareness that I've enjoyed. But many women bear a lot of stress during this time, especially caring for elderly parents: it is a cruel trick of nature.

The beginning of my story is probably quite common: I had a mother who basically pretended the menopause didn't happen. Having grown up in India, she said she enjoyed the hot flushes! But I knew her experience didn't tell the whole story. When I was in my twenties, a friend of mine told me of her own mother's 'Change of Life', as we called it back then. This strong, highly-motivated and intelligent woman experienced a dramatic change in her personality and well-being during her menopausal years. She lost all her confidence and it was very hard for her to carry on as normal. She could often be found hiding under furniture, crying and shivering. Both she and her family thought she was going mad. I think her only help from the medical world was tranquillisers. She did get through those awful days, but it terrified everyone, and things were never quite the same again.

When I was 48, I decided to go to my GP to have a check-over. I also talked to my very supportive husband. I've never been super-comfortable in my body, so for me to take an interest in this ageing process was rather confusing. I was experiencing hot flushes (which, like my mother, I rather enjoyed, except when I thought people were looking – which was pretty much never) and experimenting with a variety of alternative remedies, including black cohosh and raspberry leaf tea. I also tried lots of soya products, which I now really like! Annoyingly, I found that all the fat had snuck around to the front of my body and was now sticking on for dear life, leaving my bony bottom to fend for itself. Most unsettling!

My visit to the GP had an unexpected outcome. I was diagnosed with Lichen Sclerosus (LS), an auto-immune disease which produces white or grey itchy patches on the skin in the genital area: very unpleasant and debilitating. Little is known about it, and there is neither a cure nor adequate treatment information.

The condition generally presents – and then worsens – during menopause, but when I was diagnosed I realized that I was in fact one of the minority who had suffered from the disease since childhood. Back then I had assumed everyone had something like this but just didn't talk about it.

I told no one, not even my mother or sisters, and I felt very alone. I assumed I must either be dirty or bad or both. I tried to learn to live with it, but eventually it left me an emotional wreck. I so wish it hadn't taken me until the menopause to be diagnosed and treated.

LS is a pervasive problem and I believe it has changed the structure of my anatomy. The patches on the vulva and anus cause tiny fissures or splits in the skin (which are agony, especially when I am peeing or having sexual intercourse) and bits of the vulva become stuck together, in particular the labia, which causes changes in the physical structure of the vagina.

The disease is usually treated with topical hydrocortisone ointment: for me, this is the only thing that has really worked and it is a godsend! I always wear 100% natural underwear and use no fragrances in soap products.

The menopause still seems to me rather a taboo subject. These days we might chat about thrush or PMT, and even occasionally manage a passing comment about a hot flush or the joy of not stock-piling tampons, but it is usually spoken of in a jocular vein. Derogatory comments, from both men and women, about certain female behaviour being 'down to the menopause' are still far too common.

It really is time for a change.

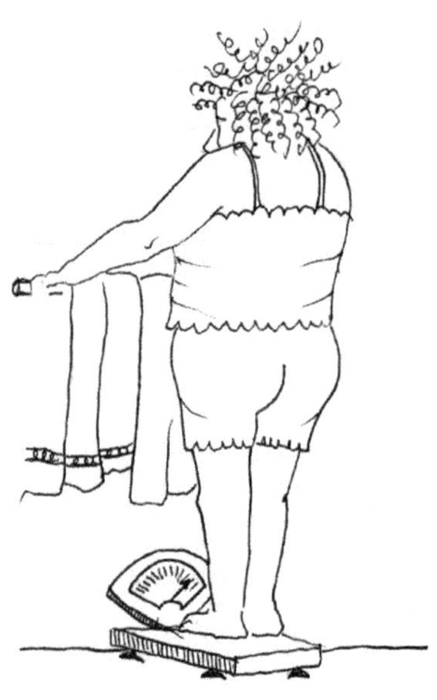

Juana's story

When I was 47, my best friend was diagnosed with a brain tumour, and died shortly afterwards. I had a period to finish all periods: it appeared nothing would stop the flow. I couldn't walk two steps without feeling the gush and seepage through my clothes, and it seemed like it lasted forever.

Putting it down to emotional trauma, I thought nothing of it...but it was the last time I would have a period.

Now, nine years on, and having heard other women's stories, I think I've probably got away with it all quite lightly. My main concerns have been the lack of vaginal lubrication during sexual intercourse and as a result the time it takes to reach (and enjoy!) full intimacy with my husband (this has crept up on me slowly, so took some time to realise), plus night sweats and the unexpected, all-encompassing, full-on hot flushes that grab me from nowhere in the most difficult-to-manage situations, such as whilst sitting in the middle row in a theatre, leaving me with a feeling of complete vulnerability, and only managed by deep breathing and 'mind over matter'.

The lubrication issue is the worst, as my husband and I always enjoyed a fun, spur-of-the-moment sex-life. I really miss those "Drop your pants!" moments! Now it needs discussion, planning and lubrication – Sylk is fabulous! Suffice to say I am extremely lucky to have such an understanding and involved husband, so we are in it together. I can't imagine how awful it would be if we didn't approach it as a united front.

I keep the night sweats under control by making sure fresh air circulates in the bedroom and having less wine in the evenings!

I know things can often be managed by HRT and I am currently close to taking some more advice about this, if only to re-tenderise my vagina!

When I was asked to contribute to this book, I thought that it would be a complete breeze: that I knew exactly how the menopause had affected me, but then I sat down with my husband and read what I had written to him. He added a few things which led to more discussion between us. The main thing he feels he has lost is the companionship in bed. I used to hate being cold in bed and would snuggle up to him for warmth, but now I can't stand him anywhere near me. Even his arm across me can cause a feeling of boiling over. This is a huge issue for him, as he feels rejected.

He also said that along with vaginal dryness, he has really noticed my lack of libido, which tallies with my thoughts on needing to 'think' about having sex, rather than just falling into it.

Interestingly, I put this discussion to my three sisters and they all claim they sailed through the menopause without even knowing they were going through it. If I felt I could, I would challenge them on libido and vaginal atrophy, but hey, they say they hardly noticed it, so what can you do?! Good for them – after all, that's what this discussion is all about...

Helen's story

"I can't possibly be old enough for this yet!" is a constant refrain inside my head these days. I still feel about 25 inside, though I do get tired more easily than I used to. Plus, a cold can wipe me out for a week, while before I would just carry on as normal. My joints ache and I feel a bit creaky first thing in the morning. Oh, and there's my complete inability to read anything smaller than size 10 font without my glasses – which my (practically teenage) optician cheerfully told me was purely age-related! My experience so far is that getting older is a pretty miserable affair.

The first sign that I might be perimenopausal was the onset of night sweats a few years ago. I would go through phases of waking up absolutely drenched in the middle of the night. There appeared to be no real pattern to this, but since I have had a Mirena coil for nine years (to manage extremely heavy periods more than as a method of contraception), I don't really have a cycle as such and rarely have what you would call a period. When I *do* have a bleed, it is usually very light and lasts only a couple of days, and then I think, "Oh yes, I suppose I *have* been a bit ratty". So perhaps that is hormone-related. I spoke to my GP about the night sweats and she told me they would probably be a lot worse if I hadn't had the coil fitted, as it releases a small amount of hormone: basically, it will help get me through the menopause.

I now have no doubt that I am perimenopausal, and I can't say I'm enjoying it at all. Aside from the night sweats, the biggest problem for me is the dreaded brain-fog. It's awful and I find it very scary. Sometimes it's so bad I worry I'm suffering from some sort of early-onset dementia or Alzheimer's. I pulled up at a set of traffic-lights last week and for a horrifying ten seconds or so had absolutely no idea where I was or which way to drive to get home. Ten seconds can seem an awfully long time when you are alone and think you are losing your mind. I struggle to find the right word for things on a daily basis. It can be anything from having difficulty with a crossword (I used to be quite good at them), to trying to write professional documents at work (I write sales proposals for a living), to attempting to remember what the thing is called to heat the water up to make myself a cup of tea...you know, a hot-water-maker-thingy...oh yes, a kettle! I get so frustrated by this because I know I am an intelligent and usually quite eloquent woman.

My teenage children think that it's hilarious how scatter-brained I have become. My son sat next to me in the car last month as we were leaving for a weekend away and asked if I was thinking about closing the front door before we left the house empty for three days: I had left it wide open and was merrily pulling off the driveway without a backward glance. I have since become somewhat obsessive about checking and double-checking locked doors.

I have recently become single again, and the break-up was so traumatic that the thought of sex is completely abhorrent to me right now. But I think that is probably more circumstantial than hormonal. Similarly, my anxiety levels have shot through the roof in the last year and I often have to give myself a talking-to just to get out of the house. The anxiety makes me feel horribly sick – but again, that may be more to do with the trauma of the break-up than with my hormones. All I know is I never used to be like this.

That's the problem. I could blame everything on my hormones, but it has been a year of such turmoil, it's hard to know where the blame really lies. About four months ago I started taking 1000mg of Evening Primrose Oil each morning for hormone-balancing, plus 1000mg of Cod Liver Oil for my poor aching joints. Oh, and I'm also taking sage. I don't know whether it's because of these supplements that things have improved, but the night sweats are now far less frequent and severe, and my mood seems to be more stable too. That is as far as I want to go in terms of treating the symptoms for the moment. I'm reluctant to go down the HRT route, as I hate taking tablets and only turn to medication as a last resort!

Ruby’s story

I passed through the menopause without too much disruption, maybe because I was very lucky and after a nine-year gap had a third child at the age of 46.

After that I was expecting that my periods would cease, and I might feel a bit different. The one symptom that I found very difficult was the hot flushes. I went straightaway onto HRT: brilliant! It felt like a new lease of life.

I stayed on that for about ten years, until they stopped producing the brand I was on. The next make was nothing like as effective, and around that time the press had scares about the link with breast cancer (which runs in my family). So I went to an NHS women's specialist. She said that hot flushes can go on for life if one stops taking HRT and suggested that being on half a tablet would be the best option: protecting the bones without risk.

So that’s what I did – and still do. I’m 74, feel fit and active, and do a lot of walking – over the Pyrenees with my son earlier this year.

Keep taking the tablets!

Clare's story

I'm 52 and in general good health. I don't smoke, I exercise regularly, I'm not overweight and I have a good diet. My only vice is dry white wine which I drink *mostly* in moderation.

Although my menopausal symptoms most probably crept up on me over a number of years, looking back it feels as if there was a time when I didn't have problems and then a time when I did.

Apart from irregular periods, I think the first symptom I noticed was hot flushes. They weren't pleasant, but I could cope. I live in an unusual street where all the neighbours are close friends. It just so happens that I'm the youngest by about ten years, so I'd been surrounded by menopausal women for a long time before any of my own symptoms began. Of all those friends, only one of them had been on HRT. The others, for various reasons, had decided to sweat it out. Whenever we got together for dinner, the back door would be opened, closed, opened, closed, as items of clothing were torn off and put back on at regular intervals.

I'd never been keen on the idea of HRT myself: I hated being on the pill when I was a teenager, and I hate taking unnecessary medicine in general, but then some other symptoms began to emerge. Suddenly, I found I couldn't concentrate. I literally couldn't gather my thoughts. I'd get confused at work and I'd have these lurches of panic: had I left the bath running? The gas on? My sleep also suffered.

At around the same time as this, sex started to become horribly painful. I found I had less and less interest in it, until eventually I had no interest at all. On top of this, the skin in and around my vagina had become so sensitive that simply wiping myself after going to the toilet would be enough to cause the skin to bleed. Soon I was in constant pain.

I went to my GP to talk about this, and she prescribed lubricants and a hormone cream, which she said I should use only for three months. The products helped while I was using them, although they were messy and unpleasant, but as soon as I stopped, all the symptoms returned. I went back to see her, and at this point she suggested I start HRT. She said I wouldn't be able to use any topical creams whilst taking HRT (this turned out to be the wrong advice) but that it wouldn't matter because HRT would help with all my symptoms.

So, almost overnight, my hot flushes stopped, my sleep improved, and I became far less muddled and confused. I still occasionally have these lurches of panic, but it's not as bad as it was. It's not that taking HRT made me feel younger, or rejuvenated, or even gave me an extra boost of energy. The way I described it at the time was that I simply felt normal again.

However, the problems I was experiencing with painful sex, specifically with vaginal dryness, got worse. My doctor referred me to a women's health clinic where I saw a consultant gynaecologist. She examined me and said I needed to apply a cream usually used for eczema. I trusted her (she was, after all, a consultant) but as it turned out she couldn't have given me worse advice. Applying the cream was like rubbing salt into an open wound. It was agony.

It was at this point, in tears almost every time I went to the toilet, that I read online about a famous menopause specialist. I made an appointment to see her privately. She was appalled at my treatment and the advice I'd received. She said that the cream I'd been given at my first GP appointment had so little hormone in it that using it for a whole year would be the equivalent of taking one HRT tablet. She gave me a stronger cream and said I could use it twice a week indefinitely with no ill effects. She also gave me another hormone treatment to use, which healed the raw, bleeding skin, plus natural vaginal moisturisers, which she said I should use at least three times a week for the rest of my life. It was the first I'd heard of them.

She said I shouldn't even think about having sex for at least three months until everything had healed and that I had to understand that this wasn't something that was going to get better without ongoing treatment. She said I had one of the worst cases of atrophic vaginitis she had seen. She also said it was no wonder I had gone off sex, and to wait and see what my libido was like once everything had healed.

That was six months ago. Everything has healed now and happily I don't have any pain. I can't say my libido is anything like what it used to be, and although my specialist did discuss the option of taking testosterone at my latest appointment, I think, for me, that's a step too far. Discussing all of this with my lovely neighbours, they joke that sex is in the past for them now. I find this so depressing. I have always had a fantastic sex life and I don't feel ready to give up on it at this stage in my life.

I suppose that if I were to sum up my experience of the menopause so far, I'd say that taking HRT has certainly helped, although I don't take it lightly, and I can't shake off the nagging doubt that I might come to regret it one day. I'm angry at how little my GP was able to help. (I actually saw three different female GPs at my practice over the course of a year and a half.) I've since found out that all the products the private menopause specialist prescribed are simply not available on the NHS as they are too expensive. My GP admitted to me that the products she first prescribed me were close to useless, but that she wasn't allowed to prescribe anything else in the first instance. This makes me angry too. Most people can't afford private medicine.

I've never felt embarrassed or uncomfortable talking about the menopause, but even so, the help wasn't there for me. I have a very supportive husband, and we're very close, but the change in our sex life has had an impact on my confidence and the way I view myself. I've seriously had to mourn the easy, pleasurable, spontaneous intimacy I took for granted for so long, even through years of infertility treatment, two babies close together in age, and other health problems we've encountered along the way.

I'm sure at some point I'll stop HRT and see how I cope: the hot flushes won't last forever. However, I do believe I'll be using the topical medicines for the foreseeable future. My body is never going to produce oestrogen again, and so if I stop the creams and moisturisers, it won't be long before my other symptoms return.

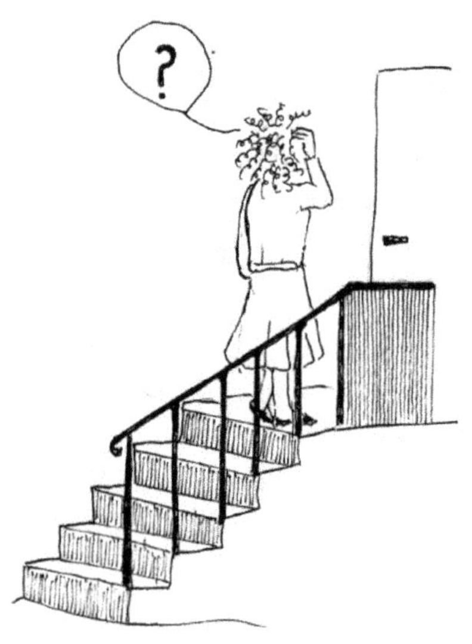

Gina's story

"That's it! He can have the children every other weekend and once during the week, but she is not to try to be their 'mum' and I am perfectly capable of raising the children on my own!"

These are the ridiculously unfounded thoughts circulating like vultures and waiting to peck away at the negative insecurities which are now an accepted part of my menopausal journey. They are the very definition of irrational: my husband is one of the most supportive and attentive partners anyone could wish for, and it would be a very brave woman indeed to take him on with five children still tugging hard at the purse strings!

But the menopause is right at the top of the list of things which challenge my mental health, from rationalising that my husband isn't having an affair, to justifying why I've put the potato peelings in the freezer (which is out in the garage). I've always been a glass-half-full girl, but for ten days a month now my irrational monkey chatters away on my shoulder and I have to work extra-hard at ensuring my thoughts and emotions are in perspective. It's a struggle, and an exhausting one, which is hard to explain and, I'm sure, hard to understand unless you are on your own menopausal journey. And with this comes the almost manic laughter and tears. Someone cracks a joke and I'm still laughing when everyone has gone home or I'm watching TV and I'm inconsolable to the injustices of life and the world.

Food. Something very close to my heart. When the children were small, I was almost obsessed with what they ate, making all their meals by hand. I would throw lunch parties for the pure pleasure of watching unsuspecting human guinea pigs taste my culinary experiments. Suddenly, this has all changed, because along with the menopause has come an inability to tolerate certain foods. Bread, pasta and all those carbohydrate staples have had to be seriously reduced in order to stop me looking seven months pregnant. As for milk…well, let's just say it has a pretty undesirable effect on my bowels. None of these food intolerances happened overnight: they have crept up on me over the past couple of years. The most lamentable loss is wine. Although I've never been a particularly heavy drinker, one glass of white at the wrong time of the month can send my heart racing and my body sweating and can result in a sleepless night where my suffering husband once again bears the brunt of my irrationality. The positive side of this is that not only have we saved a small fortune over the past few years, but my waistline and sugar intake have also been kept in check.

PERIODS! We need to get that word out there, not skirt around it with silly phrases like 'Time-of-the-month'. Let's face it, they are an absolute pain and inconvenience, and I look at my three daughters when they are moody and grumpy or scrabbling around for ibuprofen and I can't help but feel a guilty sense of relief that my time with periods (which are now heavier but shorter) is almost at an end. I think that is what keeps my irrationality in check: knowing that one day this will all settle down. The only real irritation is Gloria.

Gloria is an unwelcome guest, and she's been dragging me down physically for a couple of months. I didn't ask her to come and she has no manners, making her presence known day or night. It's just so rude. She lives in my right breast and she's hard and round but hopefully she is of a benign nature and will be leaving shortly, never to return.

And so now I find myself on another journey which is apparently often linked to the fifty-something woman trekking through the menopause, something which is outside the remits of changes in food habits and emotions. Fortunately, I found her when my rational mind was in play, but there is a nagging fear of how I will deal with this when my irrational feelings are on the rise.

As a positive person, I am fortunate enough to see all of this as an adventure, and although I'm sure there will still be some surprises in store, I am determined to wade my way through it and come out the other side mentally wiser and stronger…and preferably with a husband.

Bella's story

Hot flushes; achy joints; brain fog – I'm not that bothered with any of these. The only thing that really upsets me about the menopause is the loss of my libido, and the nightmare that comes with it: vaginal dryness.

My husband is very understanding (and possibly even slightly relieved at the sharp decrease of action between the sheets) but I've always thought of sex as the glue that binds a relationship. Go too long without it and things don't feel quite right. It's not that I'm a nymphomaniac or anything (honestly, I'm just a happily married middle-aged woman!) but I truly mourn what used to be so easy.

One side of this problem I've fixed. A pot of vaginal lubricant on either side of the bed is my wholehearted recommendation.

If only it could also restore my sex drive. Perhaps I should explore HRT options. I don't know. I'm nervous about not only the risks but also the common side-effects, and generally don't like to take medication. For me, it's all still up for debate.

Amy's story

I have always had two hormonal 'modes': Irritable Hormonal Mode and End-of-the-World Hormonal Mode. Neither is exactly pleasant, but if I had to choose between them, Irritable Hormonal Mode would win every time. I wouldn't wish End-of-the-World Hormonal Mode on my worst enemy.

My mood would often suffer in the run-up to a period when my cycle was regular. In the few days before a bleed, I would feel irritable, low and overwhelmed. I would snap at those close to me, and life would seem grey and a bit pointless. Nothing anyone did would ever help. I used to joke with my partner (afterwards!) that I might be best holing myself up in our bedroom during these episodes and having meals left outside the door. That way everyone else would be spared having to interact with someone who had temporarily lost all powers of rationality.

But I always knew (again, afterwards) that it was my hormones that were to blame, because once my period started, the fog would miraculously lift and I'd be back to my energetic, positive self. I could sense my family breathe a collective sigh of relief. No, that's a lie. I could actually hear them.

It is this that I hang onto when things go pear-shaped now. I no longer have a cycle to guide me: my periods are so irregular that I can't even begin to guess when one might put in an appearance. I've had one proper bleed in the last ten months, and two or three pathetic attempts at one (which didn't even require the use of a tampon). But I still have real emotional dips, and they feel for all the world like PMT used to, only ten times worse.

These hormonal bouts don't last long (a day or so) but are very intense, and as I said at the start, generally fall into one of two categories: Irritable Hormonal Mode (now more like Totally Furious Hormonal Mode) and End-of-the-World Hormonal Mode (now Universal Apocalypse Hormonal Mode).

Totally Furious Hormonal Mode (TFHM) usually takes the form of a blanket intolerance of anyone who doesn't pull their weight domestically. I sometimes even lash out at my partner, which is totally below the belt, since he always does his fair share of household chores. The children are a completely different matter. They're not babies anymore, and could and should do more around the house. During bouts of TFHM, they suddenly find themselves on washing-up duty, hoovering duty, tidying-their-bedrooms duty, and frankly anything-else-I-can-think-of duty. After one of these episodes, the house briefly looks like a show-home. And I swear it does the children good. They are always more appreciative of me afterwards.

Universal Apocalypse Hormonal Mode (UAHM) is something else altogether. It really is no joking matter. Thankfully, it doesn't strike very often – maybe two or three times a year – but when it does, I feel like nothing will ever be alright again. I can often be found curled up foetus-like on the bed, refusing all offers of love and help. I usually cry myself into complete exhaustion.

Occasionally, UAHM occurs in the middle of a busy work patch – and these occasions are interesting. I have never cancelled a day's work in my life – I love what I do – but if the evil hormonal fog has descended, it seriously tests my willpower to keep calm and carry on. Weirdly, the key to coping seems to be to ensure that no one else is around. If someone is there to offer sympathy, kindness or advice, it sends me further into the abyss, and I come up with multiple reasons why I shouldn't go to work/why I'm a walking disaster/why there's no point to anything. This happened last autumn. My desperate partner asked if there was anything he could do to help me, and I summoned up all of my strength and asked him to take himself off somewhere for an hour while I pulled myself together. I then went upstairs, washed my face and drove to work. When I got home that evening, the storm-clouds had magically lifted.

I could, of course, go on HRT and see if a bit of hormone-topping-up would help. But do I really want to deal with all the side-effects (and risks) when these episodes, however dreadful, are so infrequent and shortlived? Not really. I'd rather ride them out and try to remember my partner's mantra: "It's the hormones, stupid."

Alexandra's story

Puberty announced its arrival with the first of many severe migraine attacks, leaving me blind and sick for days at a time.

I had my children in my mid-twenties and after childbirth my hormones dominated my life much less. I had very regular menstruation, with what I felt was normal blood loss for four or five days, although PMT did sometimes result in emotional outbursts and unpredictable tears.

In my late thirties I began to experience much heavier blood loss, probably partly as a result of using an IUD, on medical advice as the pill was considered unsuitable. I have a strong family history of heart attacks and strokes, and in the 1980s the evidence was that the pill increased the risk. I was sterilized in my early forties, but the blood loss continued to increase. I was constantly tired and had nagging lower back pain. Social occasions were often difficult, either because I was scared to sit down on other people's furniture, or because I had ridiculously over-emotional reactions to comments or situations. At work too, I was over-emotional in my responses, collapsing in tears where I would previously have coped perfectly well.

My GP had already identified early menopause and suggested hormone patches when I was about 44. I wish I had had them earlier. They were a blessing and I wore them very successfully for five or six years. Menstrual flow was much reduced and my emotions much easier to control. I stopped using the patches as a result of forgetting to renew my prescription before going on holiday – and then discovered that I no longer had periods and felt well, happy and as emotionally well-adjusted as I was ever likely to be.

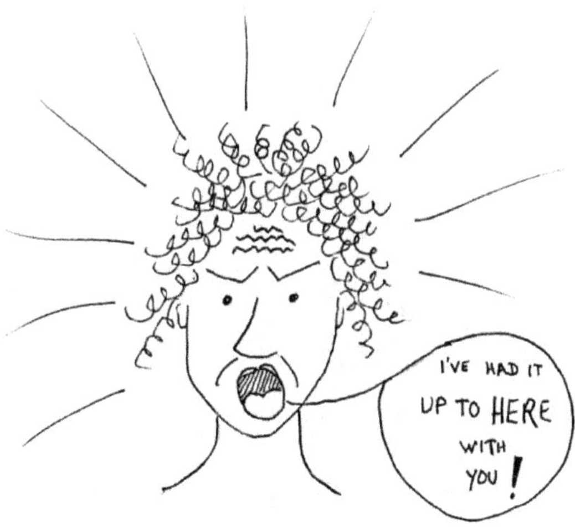

Sarah's story

I was nearly 44 when the menopause hit me. I had just been diagnosed with myeloma, bone marrow cancer, and was on my second or third cycle of chemotherapy when my periods stopped completely. There was no gentle lead-up to it: one month they were there, and the next they weren't. "Oh well," I thought, "I've got worse things to deal with!" I knew that the chemo could trigger the menopause but nobody had discussed what it would involve, so I didn't think too much about it.

I remember sitting in a friend's house three months later with the heating on, wafting myself with an old-fashioned fan. I joked about the flushes and what we have to go through as women. I didn't suffer the terrible night sweats that some people experience but I was flushing frequently throughout the day and waking up through the night because I was too hot. I would feel the sweat breaking out across my nose and forehead with no warning. Most of the time it didn't bother me but sometimes I would feel embarrassed, especially in male company, which seemed to exacerbate it.

Four years on and I still flush. I don't think it's quite as bad as it was during that first year, but I still have to think about clothing when I go out, wearing layers so that if I get too hot I can take some of them off. Now I know why women of a certain age wear cardigans: so that they can strip off whenever they flush. I tend to avoid wearing jumpers and coats because I know I will regret them later.

Before I hit the menopause myself, I never seemed to hear women talking about it – and I think that needs to change. It can be comforting to share sympathies with fellow sufferers: we are not alone in this, so why not let others know?

I have come to realise that it has had a significant impact on other areas of my life. I have always struggled with my body image, and in the last four years my whole shape has changed. Gone is my hourglass figure, as all my weight has shifted to my stomach and waist. I struggle to buy clothes because I can no longer work out what suits me. My bust has increased from a 34DD to a 34H and wearing a bra is now a painful experience. I yearn to have my old figure back and feel cheated to have this 'old lady' body at the age of 48. It has knocked my confidence and I don't feel very attractive.

In addition, my anxiety levels have rocketed and I have only recently discovered that this is actually a side effect of the menopause. My mood swings up and down like I have permanent PMT. I have had many things to deal with in the last year, including my ongoing cancer diagnosis, and it is often difficult to separate out my feelings and emotions. However, I am certain that the menopause plays a large part in this emotional rollercoaster and gives me a general feeling of not being myself.

I went to see a GP last year to see if I could get help with the anxiety. I was going through a really difficult time and felt extremely stressed. I wasn't depressed and still found joy in life, but I did feel very anxious, so I decided to try HRT. The female doctor I saw was very opposed to prescribing it. She asked nothing about what I was experiencing but insisted instead that antidepressants were a far better option: medication that would not deal with the cause and which I would have to take for a minimum of six months. I stood my ground and was given a month's supply of HRT patches. The patches wouldn't stick, so I ran out of them in three weeks and never went back for more. I felt that the brief lift in my hormone levels that resulted helped me to pick myself up and also confirmed that my emotional struggle wasn't caused solely by my inability to manage my anxiety levels.

It seems to me absolutely ridiculous that GPs are pushing antidepressants over HRT, and that there is so little discussion or recognition of the symptoms of menopause when mental health awareness has generally progressed so far. Do we feel embarrassed because the menopause is a sign of ageing? Do we feel too invisible to be seen or heard? I'm just thankful that we have each other, and that when we spot another woman fanning herself we can share a little sympathy for what is often far more than just 'a personal summer'.

Iona's story

I'd always had bad periods, ever since I started at 11. The pill helped, but they still woke me up with pain, convincing me that the world hated me, and nothing felt very real for a few days.

I was about 42, three years after I had my daughter, when they went completely AWOL. They were very irregular, anything from fourteen to forty days, and ranged from a rather pathetic pale pink splodge with almost no pain to torrential bloodbaths and searing, burning cramps from hell that kept me awake half the night and shrugged off painkillers. A thick sanitary towel and a super tampon weren't enough, and I'd frequently wake up in a wet puddle in the wee small hours. I had to master the art of cleaning up a trail of blood on the carpet from the bed to the bathroom by phone-light without waking my husband.

I also got a lot of 'fake tiredness'. I'd feel absolutely shattered and incapable of doing anything but sleep, but I'd soldier on and a few hours later I'd be back to normal. I could be jubilant one day and then have nearly a week of childbirth-level pain the next. I got into trouble at work when I let my mask slip to my useless boss. I remember saying, "You're supposed to be doing a Masters in Leadership. Do some leadership now!" I had a point – a very good one – but it didn't go down well.

A highlight happened when I was about 45. A few days earlier, I had braced myself for another onslaught when the red harbinger of doom appeared, but after a couple of days it fizzled out and I assumed I was in the clear. Assumptions are dangerous. We went to hear a friend perform at the Blackpool Opera House. We arrived about an hour early and parked some way from the theatre. As we walked, my tummy began to burn and blood started dribbling down my legs. I had nothing with me; I'd assumed my period was over. I walked like John Wayne into a café and made a wodge of loo-roll into a home-made sanitary towel, then carried on gingerly towards the theatre. A hundred metres down the street, the dams burst and blood trickled down my legs, onto my shoes and thence to the pavement. I left footprints. By now, the pain was red-hot dagger standard. It was getting late and the shops were closed. Another café, another inch-thick wodge of loo-paper. We had minutes to go before the show, and I didn't even have a plastic bag with me to protect the seat in the theatre.

Then I spotted a Pound Shop. I like Pound Shops. They have everything. The angels took pity. The Pound Shop a) was open, b) had paracetamol and c) had tampons. I told the man at the till that I loved him. I darted into the theatre loos before the show, renewed the wodge, tamponed up and glugged down the paracetamol. At the interval, I legged it to change the tampon and the wodge, and ditto as soon as the show was over.

At 47, I had a lengthy, colourful period in Australia that assaulted all of the senses (bar taste). And that, ladies, was that.

Nothing.

No nasty symptoms. No depression, anger, pain, scaly skin. Niente. The odd hot flush, but I quite enjoyed those as I hate feeling cold. Tell you what: you don't miss periods. It's been great. I'm not on HRT or anything; there's no need. I feel like it was payback for all those years of awful periods. Sweet.

Mia's story

I thought it'd be a few more years before the dreaded 'Change' reared its ugly head, but alas, it was not to be. 46: what sort of age is that to be classed as a perimenopausal woman?

My family and friends would probably tell you that I've been perimenopausal for some time. Maybe they're right.

In general, I am pretty much on the ball, but over the past few months or so, I've become increasingly forgetful. I remember feeling a bit like this when I had my daughter. As any first-time mother will tell you, sleep deprivation and general anxiety about one's parenting skills send your mind into a complete fog. The brain haze which I am experiencing now is similar, though I no longer have the excuse of getting up three times a night to feed a baby nor care what people think about my mothering abilities. I only have my hormones to blame.

Take last week, for example. I got up, showered, dressed, had breakfast, kissed my husband and daughter goodbye and walked out of the house. It was only then I realised I didn't have the car keys. I ran back to the house to collect them, but they were nowhere to be seen. I looked in all the usual places, but to no avail. I then began to panic, and screamed at everyone in my pathway, accusing them of taking my set instead of their own. Time was ticking by and I needed to get to work, so my husband thrust the spare keys into my hand and told me he'd find the lost ones once

I'd gone. Two hours later he texted me to say he'd found them in the shoes I'd worn yesterday.

Whilst out shopping recently with my mother and teenage daughter, we decided to head over to the food hall and treat ourselves to a sandwich. I was choosing what to eat when I felt a gradual build-up of heat spread through my body. It got worse and worse, until I was convinced I was going to explode. I couldn't concentrate on anything and frantically looked around to see if anyone had noticed me, and it was then that I spotted a large bucket of ice, full of bottles of mineral water. Without stopping to think, I pushed past the crowd of hungry customers, made straight for the bucket and submerged both hands in the ice. Only then did I see the look of horror and embarrassment on my daughter's face. Looking round, I saw a sea of amused faces – and at least one knowing-look from a middle-aged woman on my left. I removed my hands, wiped them on my jeans and walked away with my head held high and my blood slowly cooling down. For some time afterwards, I felt shaky and a bit unwell. My daughter suggested I eat something sweet as she thought my blood sugar levels might be low, so I wolfed down a bar of chocolate. There have to be *some* perks to this menopause business!

Olivia's story

Picture the scene: a staff room in a Further Education college, six women, aged 35 to 50, and the occasional man. In walks X, fanning herself.
"Is it hot in here?"
"No," says Occasional Man, "but I am always cold."
Thus my menopause memories begin.

Tales of hot flushes, sleepless nights, an inability to leave the house and embarrassment in public were often exchanged. I vividly remember rushing from a cab into a restaurant loo, begging to jump the queue lest I bleed out of the copious protection I had in place. Handbags had to be big enough to hold 'supplies'. Then there was a wedding ceremony in a country church I had to leave as the vows were being exchanged...no loo and no time to reach the church hall, so I crouched behind the guide hut...my handbag was small but held nothing except 'supplies'. I was back inside the church for the signing of the register, freshly plugged up and protected.

A previously regular cycle soon became erratic. The physical symptom of sore, aching limbs before a period was some sort of indicator of what was on its way and this became more intense. Then whoosh, out it all came. Question was, how was I to cope with this and continue my professional life?

A visit to the doctor resulted in a scan, blood tests and some reassurance: "This won't last forever". The scan was clear.

The blood tests confirmed that my hormones were all over the place and that I was on the verge of anaemia.
"So what now?" I asked.
"You have to do something, or there will be complications from the regular blood loss, quite apart from the tiredness you are now feeling."

HRT came to the rescue. The hot flushes stopped, I slept at night, didn't feel suddenly tearful and felt I had my life back.

Three years on I developed breast cancer. Was there a link? Possibly, but my oncologist was of the view that the benefits outweighed the risks... I am still here twenty years later, a little heavier but living life to the full.

And what about my colleagues? Three struggled through their menopauses without HRT because there was a history of associated cancers in their families, but three of us chose the chemical way out. We could stand up and teach, and attend meetings without fear of hot flushes, tears or the need to rush to the loo.

Oh, and remember Occasional Man? Well, his wife had all the symptoms too!

Abigail's story

I believe that we pass down our attitudes to our daughters when it comes to our femininity and bodies. When I was growing up, having a period was not regarded as a massive inconvenience, nor was it a reason to pull out of physical activities or have a duvet day: for me and my mother it was just a natural part of our lives – and that was before many of the more comfortable sanitary products were available. Maybe we were just lucky, but we weren't affected by excruciating pain, mood swings or heavy bleeding. And though I didn't give much thought to it at the time, I can hardly remember my mother becoming menopausal: it just seemed to be a natural progression in her early fifties, with relatively little disruption to normal life.

I thought I would follow suit, but then in my mid-forties (far too early for my liking) I started feeling weird: mood changes; hyper-sensitivity; crying for no reason; irregular periods. What was even more unexpected was the length of the perimenopausal period: in my case it was three years before my periods stopped altogether. There were no hot flushes or night-time sweats, but what came completely and utterly out-of-the-blue was The Black Dog. Full-blown, devastating, suicidal depression. It felt like that Pink Panther cartoon: wherever he walks, it's always dark and rain follows.

The hormonal imbalance knocked me for six. I honestly don't think I'd be here writing this had it not been for the total support of my GP and other local health professionals, plus SSRI medication. It upsets me to think that those years of struggle also coincided with my daughter's time at high-school. Just the other week I found a note from her, written when she was eleven or twelve. It read: "Mummy, please be happy. Turn your frown into a smile." It was hard to face the truth: that the menopause really had turned me into a different person.

Luckily, things have settled down now quite a bit, though without continuous medication and the regular practice of yoga, meditation and mindfulness, I'd be nowhere.

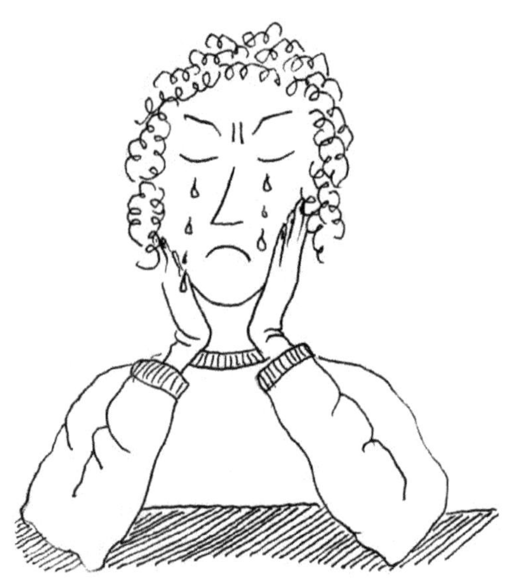

Madeleine's story

My forehead itches. Why is my forehead itchy? I have a sense of impending doom, a headache, and I can't remember words for things. Like 'hat'. "Put on your tree," I tell my 12-year-old. At lunch I tell my best friend and her colleague that I either have brain cancer or early-onset dementia. They agree: they also have brain cancer or early-onset dementia. Then we laugh: we can't all have both those things.

It must be the thing insufficiently covered in what I call 'The Woman Book'. The Woman Book covers puberty, pregnancy and birth like nobody has ever experienced those things. But The Woman Book doesn't mention 'perimenopause', the hormonal whipsaw of the decade or so before you even get to menopause. It's my midwife friend who tells me that's why I'm insane and have pimples again. And why my antidepressant has stopped working and I cry at television commercials. My belly is squishy and even though I eat well and exercise, the squish will not go. The squish is afraid I might suddenly be without food for an extended period.

I wonder whether I have ruined my children, but oops! it's too late anyway. I wonder if I should have become a marine biologist instead of a lawyer. It's definitely too late for that. I read about dolphins and wonder if I'll ever be able to retire. I used to criticize my mother for laughing in the wrong places when I told her things. I do that now and it drives my family bananas. It drives me bananas too.

On the other hand, I genuinely do not care one little bit what anyone thinks when I sing in public or go to the grocery pretty much in my pyjamas. I don't worry about people thinking I'm not smart enough. I am. This is it, what it is, who I am. I enjoy myself most of the time. I've learned things: that kindness is by far the best thing anyone can offer. I have more obligations now, but I do what I want otherwise, without having to worry about whether it's fashionable or sufficiently 'woke'. I'm both more and less tolerant than I used to be. More tolerant of ordinary foolishness; less tolerant of cruelty. I wasted so much time worrying about stupid things as a younger woman.

"Fifty-year-old woman" is how the newspaper story would describe me, whether to note an achievement or report my tragic death. Lots behind, lots ahead.

I hope!

Deborah's story

The first sign that I had started the perimenopause was the unwelcome appearance of small blistery spots in the creases by my nostrils. I was 45. I didn't have acne as a teenager (well, OK, maybe the odd pimple) but it looked like I was in for the whole enchilada now! My doctor prescribed a gel for rosacea, which worked for a few years. However, the skin on my face got a lot worse: soon I was getting blistery spots all over it. I never used to wear foundation, but it became an absolute necessity.

I investigated ways of balancing hormones through diet, which led me to try bread with various seeds in it, including pumpkin, sesame, sunflower and linseed. More recently, I have also turned to soya milk.

I have found that moisturising the skin on my whole body has made a difference. I use moisturiser every morning after showering, which has reduced itching, and apply a good quality night cream to my face. My skin has improved over the last year, but I wouldn't necessarily put it down to diet. I think I'm just at a more advanced stage of the process, so my symptoms are tailing off.

I also started getting polyps when the perimenopause started. These were mainly in my breasts (which was scary, as of course I feared cancer straightaway). I've had one polyp drained and the others just went on their own. When another showed up on a scan in my lower intestine, I went in for surgery only for them to discover it had vanished!

Horror of all horrors, I started getting cysts on my labia, usually before a period was due. I was seen by an obstetrician who didn't immediately recognise this as a symptom of the perimenopause. Thankfully, I never got as far as needing surgery. Over the last two years I have only had one. With any luck, this symptom is also on its way out.

When I last went for my cervical screening, the nurse was lovely and said she hoped that the instrument she was using to keep my labia open didn't hurt. (It didn't.) She told me that the skin there gets thin during perimenopause, which can cause discomfort, particularly if you are still having sex. I've only got two more tests to go now.

I don't think I was particularly over-emotional before I hit the perimenopause, but during the early perimenopausal years, when my periods were still regular, I suffered from extreme PMT and had sudden outbursts of anger or tears. I stopped having periods altogether for several months last year and was beginning to think it was all done and dusted…and then, lo and behold, along one came! They are now very infrequent and irregular. I started keeping a diary, so that I could be sure when I had got through a whole year without one, which is apparently when we officially reach the menopause.

Earlier this year I was diagnosed with osteoarthritis. My mother had osteoporosis, and I have been suffering with worsening lower back pain over the last seven years or so. It got so bad that it was waking me up at night. I went to the GP and was referred for an MRI scan, which resulted in the diagnosis. I now take a painkiller every night, but I think that will soon need upgrading: I've been advised that our bodies grow immune to painkillers if we take them regularly. I don't do a lot of exercise. I do a few back-presses and push-ups in the morning and have a ten-minute walk to work. I have also started walking in the evening after supper to try and help me sleep. I tried a very low dose of sleeping tablet too – and then cut that in half – but even that amount left me so switched off that one morning I nearly got run over by a group of cyclists!

HRT was not an option for me: I couldn't get on with any version of the pill as a contraceptive, so instinctively felt that I wouldn't be able to take any hormone drugs.

Sally's story

I'm 54 and can look back on the last eight years of my life like this.

During the perimenopause I kept going pretty much as normal, though it wasn't much fun. My advice to anyone would be to buy a larger handbag to accommodate supplies of tampons/towels, spare underwear, iron tablets etc – you don't know what day your period will be, and I tended to have very short cycles around this time: I suppose my body was busy getting rid of eggs.

Migraine was also part of my life at this point, so the larger handbag also needed to be stocked with appropriate tablets to cope with the sickness and headaches. Having had tummy upsets during my periods as a younger woman, I started to suffer from yet more digestive issues during the perimenopause, including rectal bleeds, for which I received excellent treatment from the NHS in the form of oestrogen pessaries.

As a professional singer, I discovered that there was less moisture in my system (which is a classic perimenopausal symptom in general) so my vocal folds weren't lubricating as effectively as before. This can actually change a singer's sound and in my case made it harder for me to sing. I soldiered on but in truth should have sought help sooner.

While all this was going on, my mother (then in her mid-eighties) was becoming more frail and needing more help.

Whereas before I would be responsible for buying birthday and Christmas gifts from my family to various relatives, I now also had to do this job for her. And also lots of other jobs. I didn't mind at the time as it was definitely helping her to keep afloat (she stayed in her own home in the north until the last few months of her life), but this all took time I didn't really have. I was already incredibly busy with both work and family (two teenage sons), and feeling constantly pushed for time brought on unpleasant physical feelings of overwhelm. My siblings were living in the USA, Germany and Derbyshire (the latter unable to travel for health reasons), so I felt that I was carrying the can in all sorts of different ways: caring for my mother; communicating with everyone to ensure we made decisions together; frequently doing the journey between London and the north.

During this time I was losing bone in my jaw and also lots of gum. I needed structural work to keep my jaw and teeth, so all my 'spare' time was spent at the dental hospital.

Throughout all this I soldiered on, never daring to give in and take a day off work. I was afraid of being thought of as weak, so didn't dare to admit that I was a woman with hormones. Looking back, I should have taken time off to care for my mother. I consider it significant that my periods stopped at the time when she was most unwell.

Since then, what has changed? Well, I am now better able to dress as a woman (having previously dressed in a less feminine way, I now enjoy my curves more). Physically, I'm possibly more confident but at the same time have lost some strength. Yoga is great at helping me to regain my poise, and so is a top-up course of Alexander Technique lessons. I have really wonderful female friends who have nurtured me (as I nurture them) and we run together most weeks. I now freelance as a choral conductor, singer and singing teacher, and feel greater ownership of my body than previously. I know that eventually it will let me down, so I'd best enjoy this time of my life while I can.

So here I am! I consider myself lucky in many ways: I have a husband and two healthy sons, I enjoy my work and I am on good terms with friends and family. But the path to this has not been exactly easy!

Tamsin's story

Just before my 50th birthday I was found to have an ovarian cyst. Clearly, there was a concern over whether this was benign or malignant, and therefore I was persuaded to have an urgent total hysterectomy. Before this I was having very regular periods which were neither heavy nor troublesome. My hormone profile showed the early signs of perimenopausal change, but other than that it was unremarkable. I was naturally upset at the prospect of losing not only my uterus but also both ovaries.

During the operation, a replacement hormone pellet was inserted into my abdomen. This must have been a 'one-size-fits-all' and my hormone levels shot up well above normal levels, possibly because I am relatively small and slim. This produced very unpleasant symptoms of pelvic burning, sore breasts, disturbed sleep pattern and erratic emotions. I think it was about three months before the hormone levels returned to 'normal'. The cyst turned out to be benign.

I was then started on hormone replacement patches (oestrogen only) and these I continued for nearly six years. I had no symptoms and was very happy with this form of HRT. Unfortunately, at a routine mammogram I was found to have a lesion, which on biopsy turned out to be a high grade multifocal ductal carcinoma in situ of my right breast. I had a total mastectomy, and because the tumour was oestrogen-sensitive, I was advised to discontinue my HRT. I did then experience some menopausal symptoms. I became much more tired at work and my muscles often felt very achy and sore. These were my main worries, as I was still working in a demanding role and sometimes had to force myself to be active and smiley! My brain also seemed to be more sluggish and I felt suddenly much older. I had some night sweats but these were infrequent and quite mild compared with those experienced and described by my friends. My sleep was disturbed once more. I never had any hot flushes in the daytime. I did get more cystitis symptoms but I have always been susceptible to urine infections, so it is difficult to know if this was purely a hormonal effect.

I discussed my symptoms with my very approachable breast surgeon and together we agreed to restart the oestrogen patches which had suited me so well in the past. These provided instant relief and I was soon back to my bouncy, energetic self. However, it was agreed that this treatment should not go on indefinitely, and after a further four or five years it was decided that I should aim to discontinue HRT. I didn't stop the patches straightaway, but very gradually reduced the dose that my body was receiving, firstly by changing the patches less frequently and then by cutting the patch in half and finally in quarters. I don't know if this is an acceptable or orthodox method but it suited my body very well and apart from a little sleep disturbance and a few night sweats I had no other major symptoms. I did experience some vaginal dryness, which I treated with local creams.

I was fortunate to have firstly a female gynaecologist and then a male breast surgeon, both of whom were very easy to talk to and who communicated well with me as a patient, especially the breast surgeon. Now I am through this time, the only problems that remain are vaginal dryness, which I treat with tablets; some osteoporosis of my spine, for which I take vitamin D and calcium tablets (plus I try to remain active); a rather poor sleep pattern, which has persisted; and, more annoyingly, recurrent urinary tract infections, for which I am undergoing further investigations. It is now twenty years since my mastectomy and I am enjoying a fulfilling retirement.

Emily's story

I can liken my journey through the menopause to a snake shedding its skin: extraordinarily painful during the process but emerging transformed in ways that I would not have thought possible.

I had just turned 50 when the menopause started to kick in, and I'd say it had an impact on me both physically and emotionally. My mother, whom we had nursed through her cancer, died in the September of that year. I then discovered that one of my ovaries had a tumour and I was advised that both ovaries should be removed. Added to this, the management of the school in which I had taught for ten years started bullying me. Needless to say, this had absolutely nothing to do with the quality of my teaching and everything to do with finance. It was like a triple-whammy hitting me all at once.

On the physical side of things, I didn't suffer too much in the way of hot flushes, and I think that regular exercise helped with this. It was emotionally that I suffered the most, trying to come to terms with my mother's death and being told on a regular basis that I was a useless teacher. My confidence was at rock bottom and this in turn affected my energy levels.

I was faced with a stark choice: to take the school to court or to leave. My confidence was so low that I couldn't face the idea of a court case, so I came up with another plan. For several years I had been writing art history books for children's art projects and I began to wonder whether I could persuade a school to let me teach art part-time, allowing me more time for my writing. Amazingly, I succeeded and found a position at a boys' school: a baptism by fire, since I'd never taught just boys before.

Four years on, I have been offered a permanent position and am absolutely thrilled.

I think my advice would be to accept the transition into menopause and see it as a chance to re-evaluate your life, try out new things and keep challenging yourself.

Nicola's story

I don't remember exactly when the symptoms started: probably in my mid-to-late forties. Mostly, they involved occasional hot flushes – or, as a colleague used to call them, 'short, personal holidays in the tropics'!

I was teaching IT Applications at a Further Education College, and being immured in a room with twenty-one computers going full blast in the middle of summer was not conducive to being cool, even at the best of times. I wore the lightest of cotton dresses, and frequently contemplated going home to change. It got to the stage where I would take a change of dress, top and underwear with me. Bras chafed, as did damp pants – urrggh! I can still feel areas of skin beneath my boobs where chafing occurred. Even when the winter months came around, I would bring spare clothing with me, as I didn't know when the dreaded tropical holidays would strike.

This was combined with irregular periods, which had lost their previous clockwork sometime after motherhood. Because of this irregularity, I kept a diary to give me a rough guide as to when I might expect one, and knowing that menopause was pending, I tried to analyse what was going on with my body, though not terribly successfully!

I can't particularly remember any emotional problems, unless by any chance you count leaving your husband for ten years! Is homicide a symptom of the menopause? Hmmm!

I had my last period five months after my 54th birthday. I think I had a pretty good deal, because although the hot flushes returned occasionally, as I write aged 64, I haven't had one for a number of years.

Incidentally, my older sister and I both had terrible trouble with period pain in our youth, to the extent of losing whole days as martyrs to it (pain relief not being as advanced when we were young: it was aspirin or nothing). We also experienced morning sickness with our pregnancies, which our younger sister thought was all in the mind! This sister had very few problems with periods and passed through pregnancy easily, but, boy, did she suffer through the menopause!

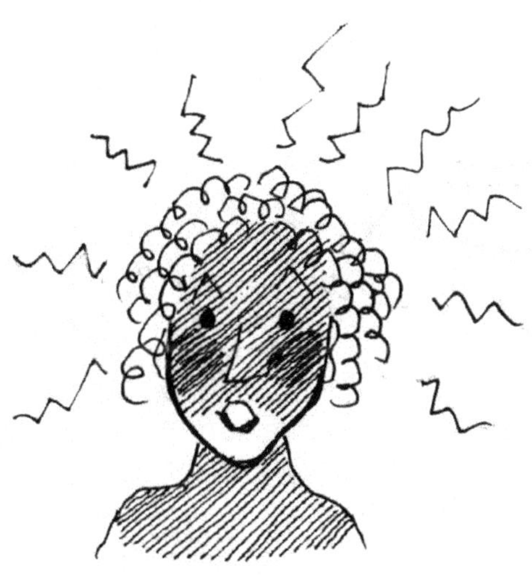

Ursula's story

I would describe my experience of the perimenopause as being somewhat like the Ancient Mariner, lost at sea with a number of albatrosses clinging to my neck. Now, at 53, I'm hoping I'm nearly through with it.

I started my journey around the age of 45 with the onset of very heavy periods, although I didn't really have a clue what was going on. It also coincided with a period of depression and the sense that my life had suddenly been turned upside-down.

A visit to the doctor resulted in antidepressants and the comment, "I'm sorry, I don't do periods. You'll have to consult a female doctor for that." I was determined to get off antidepressants and took them for around eight months, using yoga and music to reach the point where I felt confident enough to manage without them. My husband and I also went to Relate, as we thought we needed to re-establish our relationship and have more fun after the long years of being mainly parents.

However, this began a time of redefining my sense of self: my children were sitting GCSEs and A levels and planning their futures, but I had no idea what my future was.

My perimenopause ran alongside my husband being diagnosed with two types of cancer and my sister having breast cancer. My daughter left home to go to university, which I found very hard as I had spent a lot of time with her and hated the idea of being stuck at home: just me and a pair of blokes. It took a while to appreciate how nice having my son and my husband all to myself actually was.

In short, it was a period of many losses and changes.

Through it all, I have been fortunate in getting back to my singing and meeting a lot of new people through my music, and this has been the rock upon which I have rested. I have also practised yoga and meditation for many years, both of which have been hugely valuable tools during times of emotional upheaval.

I find it difficult to separate the emotional effects brought on by the physical changes in my body (such as the itching skin, the aching joints, the weight gain and the indigestion) from the emotional effects caused by the changes in my family life. But looking back, I am very glad to be here at this stage in my life with my children doing so well, my husband healthy and many things to look forward to.

The middle years are certainly a challenge, but now I'm through what I think is the worst of it and things are beginning to settle down, I'm looking forward to improving my fitness, losing the weight I've put on and forging ahead with new projects and plans. Spending more time with my elderly mother is also now important as she becomes less able to cope.

The perimenopause has been a very turbulent time for me, but the thing to remember is that it does end, things do calm down and we emerge with much more inner strength and insight into ourselves, and as a consequence more understanding and sympathy for those who struggle with difficulties in their lives.

Carrie's story

My family tend to get very old, or not very old at all. My grandmother lived into her second century: it was her proud boast that she had seen six monarchs on the British throne (even though she had no recollection of Victoria), as had all fifteen of her cousins. I remember going to the funeral of one who died at 87 (he was a lay preacher and also a drag artist, which is another story altogether) and seeing the sad headshaking of a table full of robust near-centenarians lamenting his untimely death, cut down in his prime. But one 'never-was-a-great-uncle' died at the age of 20 from consumption, and several died in infancy. The message to me, growing up amongst a very large extended family, was clear: if you make it past 21, you will probably be propping up the pillars of the temple for a very long time.

Whether because of or despite this, I tend to forget I am now old. What's 50, 51, 52 in the grand scheme of things? I still feel more or less the same as I did when I was 21, even if a mad-haired old bat has taken up residence in the bathroom mirror. Most of me works. My son may have totalled my internal workings on his way out into the world (and my daughter followed the same way a couple of years later) but the rest of me feels, if I'm honest, in better nick than when I was as fresh as a daisy (except I never was).

My boobs arrived overnight when I was 12, popping out like some sort of outsized joke. For the next ten or twenty years, I basically just gangled about, crashing into things both metaphorically and literally. I fell in love with a lot of people, mostly hugely more attractive than I was, and who were generally horrified when my roving and randy eye fell upon them. I didn't work hard enough. I met my husband, and to my lasting astonishment, instead of running away in horror when he caught me perving at his legs, he turned up with a bag of fudge and an invitation to go and see *Chicken Run.* We got married, had two children (I nearly died in the attempt) and settled down to poddle our way through middle age and retirement. My job worked out, developed, changed, and to my surprise I found I had a family and something that passed for a career.

And then, one morning that in my excessively punctual cycle should have been D-day, nothing happened. I knew I wasn't pregnant, my husband having been in Glasgow for the entire month and me having enjoyed undisputed possession of the duvet. As I could normally set my watch by it, I was a little bit surprised, but not unduly concerned: everyone skips a period every now and then, surely? But then I had my first hot flush, and my tranquil nights became punctuated by several changes of nightwear as I woke up soaking and stressed. My hormones don't do things by halves. Puberty had arrived like a tombstone dropped from a hot air balloon, and so did the menopause. But it was mercifully quick. For five months I sweated, and large chunks of my system turned off: I felt as though the night-watchman had woken up with a start and realised he had left everything running, tearing about randomly pulling out plugs until the machines all fell silent.

And the silence was deafening. The decision about whether or not to have a third child was suddenly not even on the table. I found some grey hairs. I still enjoyed sex but wasn't that bothered if my husband was already snoring when I came to bed. The cheerful distant lust I had enjoyed for a couple of my colleagues was no longer even interesting. And there was the knowledge that, even if I clocked up my ancestors' impressive lifespans, the odds were that I had lived more years than I had yet to live, and that I really ought to bear that in mind. My family tend to drop dead rather than slowly decline, and although the clock had always been ticking, in the sudden quiet I found I could actually hear it.

But I could hear something else too: my own voice. I love my job. I now do lots of things I would, ten years ago, have shied away from because it wasn't the time. Well, now there isn't going to be another shot. I conduct. I write. I sing. I've decided not to colour my hair. We have a lot more sex (though admittedly somewhat carefully, because there are several members of my family who only exist because the old ovaries fired off one last round) because – well, because why not? We only live once. I've even recovered the joys of long-distance lust, even if these days it is a twinkle in the eye rather than a raising of the pulse.

Do I miss being young? Yes. I miss my joints not creaking. I miss looking fresh. I miss being thinner: my metabolism definitely gets slower by the day. I miss the possibility of having more kids, even if I never took it. I miss planning for a longer future. But there is so much I don't miss. My sanitary towels are waiting for my teenage daughter to require them. I love not having to deal with them myself. I love not having to remember to check my handbag for migraine tablets every day, since my bimonthly migraines died with my cycle. I love being able to wear white. And I care so, *so* much less what other people think. Do I have a beach body? No. Do I take my body to the beach? You bet. Do you think I'm attractive? No? Well, sod off then. And don't pat my backside, or I'll have your arm off.

Now, beyond what's out of my control, things happen on my own terms. Offer me a good job and I'll still jump at the chance, though I won't pass up going to my daughter's Christmas concert for it. And perhaps I won't go and network at that party tonight: I'd rather put my feet up and watch *Casualty*. I'm still an ambitious professional: just not at any price. Something about losing my youth has given me a determination to make the most of the years I have left. After all, if I follow family tradition, I'm only halfway through.

The Men

Harry's story

Men experience the menopause twice in their lives. Not as physical changes within themselves, but as surprising (and occasionally hilarious) Jekyll-and-Hyde-style changes of personality in the two women they are closest to: their mothers and their wives.

My mother adopted me when she was 40. She was a truly passionate tigress of a mum, and it suited us both very well. I loved her ability to scoop me up in her arms and wrap me close whenever I was upset or anxious. If anyone came near to threatening me, child or adult, she would be in their face: either physically jousting with them, or using words to pierce their hearts.

I was subjected to threats at school on a daily basis. On one memorable occasion, my mother heard someone shouting at me, "Give me your lunch money or I'll rip out your kidneys!" She turned the (largeish) boy around, threw him against the fence and leaned into him: "Touch my child again and I'll cause you such pain you will become a vegetable, and your arms and legs will shrink and turn black!" She then rested her beautifully manicured nails on his face, applied a fair amount of pressure, and screamed, "Do you hear me?" I was 7; he was 8. He ran away as fast as his legs could carry him, and no one ever tried to steal my lunch money again.

At first I thought my mother's behaviour was normal – I knew no different – but everyone else at school saw her as utterly unhinged. I remember overhearing a young mum talking in hushed tones: "So sad for such a little boy to have to deal with a mother going through The Change."

Once I realised this sort of behaviour wasn't normal, it was rather disconcerting to see my mother – a funny, bright and very rational woman – turn into a paranoid, hysterical, screaming banshee. I remember my father once forgetting to buy bread for the bread sauce, and World War Three breaking out. My mother burst into tears, fell to her knees, threw her head back and screamed that he hated her, that we couldn't possibly eat chicken without bread sauce, and that he never did what he was asked to do, even after nineteen years of marriage. My father – a gentle, quiet and loving man – dropped the post he was glancing through and walked out of the front door. I stood there, mesmerised by my mother who was still raging: pulling at her hair, screaming incomprehensible words, and banging the kitchen floor with her fists. When the front door shut behind my father, she stopped, got to her feet, walked to the stove and stirred the gravy. Ten minutes later my father and the bread arrived home. My mother didn't even look at him: she reached out and he placed the loaf into her hand. There were no words. My father shot a quizzical look in my direction, which I returned. The silence drained every morsel of warmth from the room. My mother continued to prepare dinner, and when it was ready the plates landed a little too loudly on the table. We ate in an unbreathable vacuum of silence. My mother waited until my father and I had finished, and then she got up and very quietly announced that she was going to bed.

I have hundreds of similar stories, which span at least twelve years. As I got older, my father and I would go shopping together and he would explain that my mother was going through what was called 'The Change of Life'. Apparently, she was not certifiably insane, and I should rest assured that after her outbursts she would always return to her normal, loving self. During the moments when she was definitely *not* herself, we should learn not to engage with her directly, but offer tea and biscuits, until such time as she would take herself to bed. I thought this was good advice, and it comforted me to know that there was an explanation.

By the time my mum reached her fifties, I had become a hormone-ridden teenager. Every now and then I would forget the 'don't engage' rule, and on these occasions my mother would reach for the nearest available object and hurl it in my direction. I would retaliate with my own object. This would go on until the screaming reached fever-pitch and the objects created holes in the walls, and then my mother would run crying to her bedroom and lock the door. My father would come home to a version of Coventry after The Blitz. (Incidentally, when my parents eventually passed away within two weeks of each other, and I was packing their lives into boxes, I noticed that they had very few *objets d'art* in their lives: my mother and I had previously made an excellent job of clearing the decks.)

Something changed when my mother turned 55. Once a few objects had been thrown, she would start to laugh, and then we would both end up writhing about on the floor in hysterics. It was really rather miraculous.

When my wife started to become upset over seemingly small things in her middle years, an increasingly noisy bell rang in my head. At least now I could turn to the internet for advice.

She explained what was going on with her, and we began to drink soya milk (initially a horrible experience, but one I grew to love). This, together with a mixture of seeds ground into her breakfast each morning, and a variety of herbs, seemed to help with her moods.

Her hot flushes would end up with me drowning in all the bedclothes, often unable to breathe as some garment or other was flung over me. The herbs did wonders for this, but we did have to give in to single duvets, so that when warm occasions struck, she could throw the cover onto the floor, rather than me.

It was important to us both that this enormous change in my wife's life was experienced as much as possible together, rather than as something she simply had to endure on her own. I learnt that throwing objects just led to tears and even more hysteria: kindness, warmth and understanding were all that was necessary. This took quite a lot of bravery on my part: it's pretty hard to get near someone who is very upset and angry, and harder still to remain kind. A bitter retaliation of words never helped: in this state my wife had uncharacteristically Thesaurus-like powers of dark and hurtful invective.

We came up with our own solution, which was called 'Embrace the Exploding Bomb'. It came from the idea that embracing an exploding bomb meant that you were spared pain. So when I saw my wife getting into a terrible state, I would take a deep breath and hold her in my arms. There was often a struggle and lots of demands to "Get off!" or "Go away!" but eventually the dam of tears would burst and she would relax in my embrace and the world would look better.

Oh, and I have a rather more sophisticated take on my father's offerings of tea and biscuits. I prefer to make my wife a soya latte with a shot of black cohosh.

Jamie's story

In my opinion, men haven't got the first clue about the menopause. We're not told anything except "I'm on The Change" or "It's my age" or "I'm having a flush". Perhaps it's why we have sheds – they can't only be for storage.

It's like Jekyll and Hyde: one minute your wife's normal, and then she's away with the fairies. I just tell the kids to keep their heads down, because if anyone dares argue with her, they'll always lose.

Mind you, with three daughters in the house, hormones are constantly flying around, so you soon get used to it!

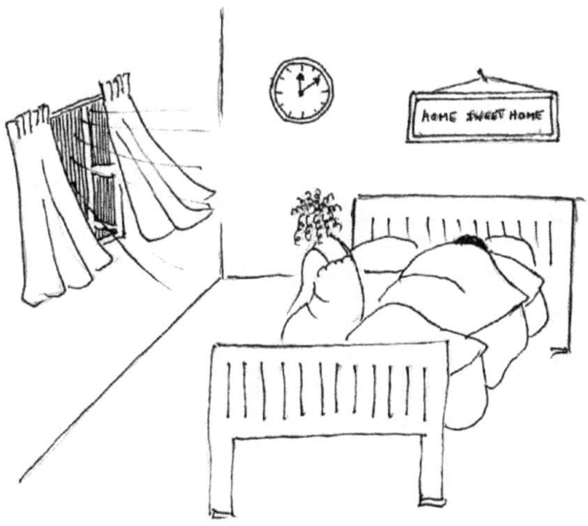

Omar's story

I had known my wife for about two years before our relationship started. During the previous eight years, I had managed both a disastrous marriage and a completely sterile relationship: quite an achievement on my part.

The new relationship grew very gently. I felt a previously-forgotten (or maybe even totally-unknown) warmth for this woman and knew we were going to end up in bed together…and frankly I was scared. But it happened and I cannot forget the joy and wonderful rightness of our intimacy. She had a healthy and uninhibited libido – sex for her was such a natural thing – whereas I was cramped and suppressed. But her warmth and affection drew me out of that (although at first she tended to take the lead). It felt like being welcomed home after a very long journey.

Marriage and children followed, and our loving physical relationship continued unabated. There were emotional upsets, but I soon realised these followed a predictable hormonal pattern. I took to marking my diary with little red asterisks to warn me one might be due!

Time passed and we became busy with the demands of daily life, children and our careers. By now my wife was in her mid-forties, and her emotional upsets started to become more pronounced and our lovemaking more sporadic. Whilst it sometimes looked as if external causes were to blame, it became clear that the onset of the menopause was vastly exaggerating things. We kept the lines of communication open at all times, and that made all the difference.

Nearly a quarter of a century on, we love each other more than ever. As for the physical side of our relationship, there's nothing that a little vaginal lubrication and a helping hand can't solve!

Stefan's story

Male perspectives on the menopause are as rare as hens' teeth. This is the woman's domain, the sufferer's domain – and I use that word advisedly, whilst recognising that there are many women whose experiences are benign or even asymptomatic. Brave is the man who ventures any opinion less than entirely sympathetic. Woe betide the man who suggests it has affected him too. The territory is dangerous because it falls into a similar category to PMT and childbirth. Men cannot directly experience either, so their views are unwelcome. There is a thin line between reasonable comment and perceived sexism that most men would be hesitant to cross. But perhaps this is odd. Direct experience is not a precondition for comment in most spheres. The genius of this book is its collation of both male and female opinions about the menopause. It recognises that there is a place for a male voice in a full understanding of this bodily and emotional process.

Nothing I say detracts from the impact that the menopause can have on the woman herself. The male experience will, and should, always take second place to the direct sufferings of the afflicted woman. I have strayed again into the language of illness because that is its closest parallel. Sleeplessness, emotional instability, night sweats, hot flushes. When these symptoms persist with no end in sight, misery and discomfort ensue.

It would be naïve to think that the life of the whole family is not adversely affected under these circumstances. At its worst, the menopause unsettles its foundations. Transient ill-temper is easy to ride out, but when it persists, day after day, it can be much more corrosive. When I faced irrational anger and irascibility regularly, I found it difficult to maintain sympathy. Too often I would bite back, either to defend myself or to plead an injustice. Unsurprisingly, these responses would not always go down brilliantly. And I was probably hugely irritating myself anyway.

There were times when I wondered whether my wife had had a personality transplant. I was fortunate to find her turn a corner emotionally after a number of months and rediscover her old self, even if she still glowed and sweated at unwelcome hours.

I wouldn't wish the menopause on anyone, woman or man. It's not exactly a learning experience to be welcomed. And what have I learnt? What might a man best do to help himself and his partner? Well, sympathy for her physical symptoms is essential. One might try to avoid emotional instability by upping one's game and giving no cause for discontent. However, this is hardly realistic and certainly impossible to sustain. Understanding, communication and pulling one's weight are the only practical antidotes.

Emil's story

My wife and I are both in our early sixties and have never once spoken about her menopause. We don't really talk about personal stuff.

Looking back, there were definitely times in the last ten years or so when she was moodier than usual: sudden outbursts of irrational anger and, on one memorable occasion, a terrible "What have I done with my life?" weeping session, but these episodes were quickly brushed under the carpet.

To be honest, I think we've been drifting apart for years, so if she did have any hot flushes or other physical symptoms, I didn't notice them. Maybe our relationship has never been quite right. Certainly, since our daughters left home, it has felt awkward even being in the same house as her.

Writing this makes me a bit sad. Perhaps things would have been different if we'd opened up to one another and communicated more, but it's too late for that now.

Oliver's story

After a number of relationships – and now a very happy marriage – I have had much experience of hormone-related mood-swings. Those associated with PMS can often be upsetting, but pale into insignificance when compared with the wild outbursts of the menopause. My normally warm, loving and gentle wife can, on occasion, turn into a raging, inconsolable and totally unrecognisable monster. Fortunately, these outbursts are infrequent, and as our relationship is strong, we cope with them pretty well, though they can be briefly terrifying.

What follows is an example of just one bad day, which erupted inexplicably in the middle of a period of otherwise unalloyed domestic contentment.

A Sunday in November:

Act 1: 10am

Me: What's wrong, darling? Something's getting to you. Come on, what is it? It's always better to share problems.

Her: I don't matter to you anymore! I might as well not be here! You'd be better off without me, then you could do all the things you used to, like going to the pub with your friends. You'd have a stress-free life and enjoy yourself.

Me: Have you forgotten that I love you and chose to be with you? This is what I want.

Her: And what's happened to our physical relationship? We don't seem to have sex much anymore.

Me: We had it last Sunday afternoon, and I've been working away since then. We can't have sex by text. Is this some sort of phantom ovulation? Does your body want to be pregnant again?

Act 2: 2pm

Her: I know you love me really. It's just that you don't show it.

Me: I have very deep feelings for you, but they can get suppressed by practicalities. We can both get exhausted and libido-less. There are demands everywhere, but we do have times of mutual passion, which you seem to forget.

Her: I'm a total let-down! I should cancel all my work and acknowledge what a mess I am!

Me: This is just your hormones talking. Don't be silly.

Her: Shut up! Don't tell me not to be silly! Go away! I want to be alone!

Act 3: 7pm

Her: I'm sorry. I do love you really. I just felt awful earlier: I don't know why.

Me: Bloody menopause! But I knew it was that and that it would pass. I think I need to put my arms around you. There. Better?

Her: Yes. Sorry.

Me: Sorry not allowed. Might be nice to check on the libido though.

Her: That would be lovely.

<u>Curtain</u>

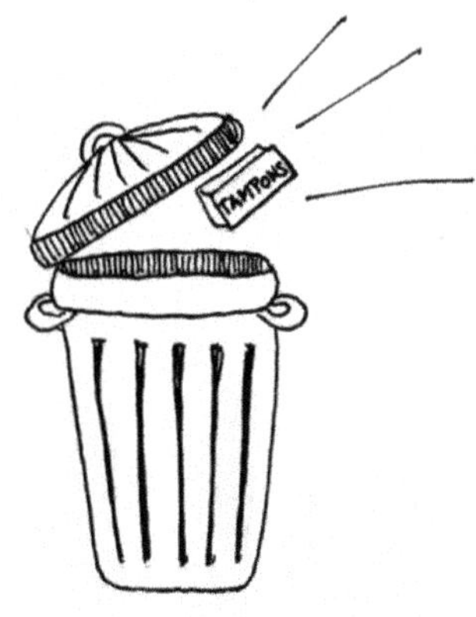

Coming soon...

The Menopause Monologues II

If you've enjoyed reading this book and would like to share *your* story (anonymously, unless you would prefer otherwise), please send us a direct message through our Facebook page (*The Menopause Monologues*). We'd love to hear from you!

Thanks

…to Joseph, for his unwavering (if uncharacteristic) patience.

…to Emily, for putting up with him.

…to Gabriel, Naomi, Marianne, Janine, Esther and Kate, for their advice and encouragement.

…to Nick, without whom the compiler of these stories would have been washed away in a tsunami of hormones and hot flushes many moons ago.

www.ingramcontent.com/pod-product-compliance
Ingram Content Group UK Ltd.
Pitfield, Milton Keynes, MK11 3LW, UK
UKHW020416250726
13967UKWH00007B/2676